ersus-Host Disease

itis

Syndrome

undrome

19/04   9:05 AM   Page 11

us System Toxoplasmo

an Disease, or Relapsing

19/04 9:05 AM Page 16

smitted Urethritis

19/04 9:05 AM Page 17

ioracic Aortic Aneurysi

inemia Due to Dapsone

With Pulmonary and

erebral Artery Occlusio

ease

yndrome

gmentosum

ain Spotted Fever (RMS

se

nduced Phototoxic Dern

eimer Reaction

ase (Thromboangiitis (

osure

Syndrome With Necrol

rome

ilis

(Xanthoma Palpebraru

ome

aused by Arsenic Toxici

ycosis

nentosa

tanea Tarda

er's Cust

is

drome

ilis

ise (Hepatolenticular De

ipid Antibody Syndrom

igricans

1) Cryoglobulinemic Vas

of Queyrat

itoma

mic Amyloidosis

ta

drome

ongue (Lingua Nigra)

t (Neuroarthropathy)

ıl Scalded Skin Syndron

sen's Disease)

laris

Syndrome

ar Hypertrophy

plexy

Myocardial Infarction an

ntinued): Evolution of

inued): *Evolution of An*

is

(Chigger) Bites

ion

ciency Ulcer

on Syndrome (SJS) and

ongue, or Benign Migrat

drome

Cholesterol Emboli, or

ia Due to Valve Hemol

ertensive) Ulcer or M

losum

sociated Fever

ced Thrombocytopenia

e Distal Long Biceps Te

ariasis and Bancroftial

neurusm

tosis Type 1

iterranean Fever (FMF,

Still's Disease

on-White Pattern

Nodosa

lein Purpura

ict Dermatitis (Rhus D

ciated Diseases

cardial Infarction

ium

Pseudomonas *Nail Infe*

tadenoma

morrhagic Telangiectas

arathyroidism

mochromatosis

Myocardial Infarction

Dissection in Marfan S

rcinoma

Joint Disease (Osteoart

1e Liver

ease

y Anemia

roid Cancer

1 Tick Paralysis

e (**Loxosceles reclusa,** *o*

Pseudotumor in Wegen

y Syndrome

Imperfecta

kin Reaction

cuminata (Genital War

philis

viation

Gonococcal Infection

iritis (Arthritis Mutilan

al Sarcoma Causing Hy

jtoma

alsy

ripheral Gangrene

mic Amyloidosis With

Intravascular Coagulo

us Erythematosus

ubitus) Ulcers

mochromatosis

nd Mouth Disease

oides or Cutaneous T-C

Deformity

Teeth of Congenital Syp

hangitis Due to Mycob

idrome

rpetiformis

low

inulomatosis

tis

ıl Toxic Shock Syndrom

ltiforme

initis (in setting of Reit

is

ngrenosum

enomenon (Superimpo

Stroke

emia

Associated With Angiot

litis

se

Cava Syndrome

se of the Breast

Atrioventricular Block

ia

r (Arterial Sclerotic Oc

Arthritis

5/18/04 12:50 PM Page 319

mia

ome

S

Ulcer

uloma

ri-Harada Syndrome

gioma

rcinoma

ipoidica Diabeticorum

ctiosum (Fifth Disease)

XII *Palsy*

ry Cirrhosis

APPENDIX

Endo)

etal Diseases (Musc)

s (Vasc)

INDEX

, 161
dies, 262

8:10 AM   Page 355

45, 143
lossitis 133

8:10 AM   Page 357

, 257

5, 325

etic acid, 67

8:10 AM   Page 361

141

8:10 AM   Page 362

. 319

8:10 AM Page 363

stimulating hormone), 199
oma, 179

8:10 AM   Page 364

y, 237

8:10 AM   Page 365

m, 33, 285

8:10 AM Page 368

Ioma 259